Mediterranean Diet Handbook for Beginners:

Full Guide on Mediterranean Diets; How It Works Plus Its Benefits; What to Consume& Comparisons with Other Diets; Meal Plan For a Whole Week& So Much More

By

Doctor Peter L. Turnbull

Copyright@2020

TABLE OF CONTENTS

THE END....................................62

CHAPTER ONE

INTRODUCTION

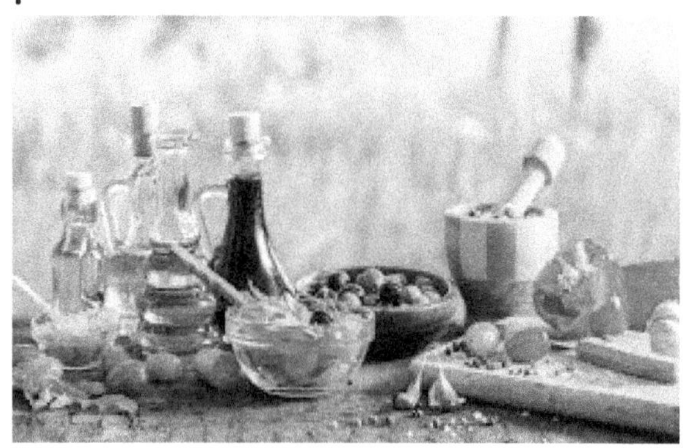

The Mediterranean eating routine depends on the customary nourishments that individuals used to eat in nations like Italy and Greece in 1960s.

Scientists noticed that these individuals were particularly sound contrasted with Americans and had a generally safe way of life with regards tocontracting certaininfections or ailments. **And**

this was as a result of their healthy meals or diets.

Various investigations have now indicated that the Mediterranean eating routine can cause weight reduction and help forestall coronary failures, strokes, type 2 diabetes and sudden passing.

This guide portrays the dietary example ordinarily endorsed in contemplates that propose it's a solid method of eating.

Consider the sum of this as a general guideline, not something written in stone. The game plan can be adjusted to your individual needs and tendencies.

The Essentials

Consume: natural items, vegetables, seeds, vegetables, nuts, potatoes, breads, flavors, flavors, fish, whole grains, as well as olive oil (extra virgin).

Eat with some limitation: Poultry, eggs, cheddar and yogurt.

Eat just rarely: Red meat.

Make an effort not to eat: Sugar-improved rewards, included sugars, arranged meat, refined grains, refined oils and other significantly dealt with sustenance.

CHAPTER TWO

FOODS TO AVOID PLUS THE ONES TO CONSUME AS WELL AS THE DRINKS TO GUZZLE

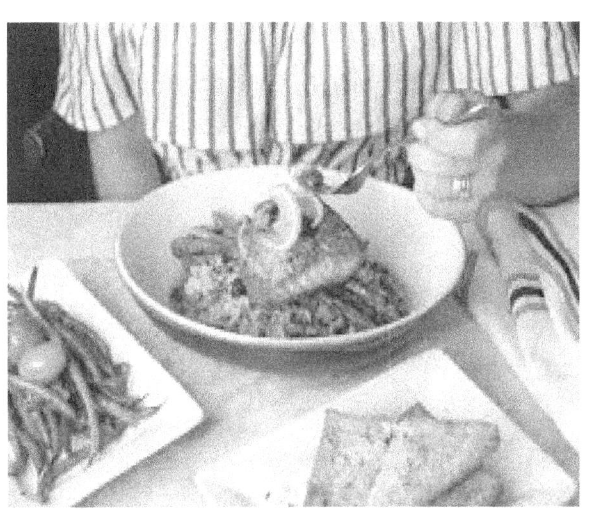

Keep up a key good ways from these unhealthy foods

You should keep up a key good ways from these bothersome sustenance and trimmings:

Built-in sugar: Soda, sweets, solidified yogurt, table sugar and various others.

Grains that are refined: Pasta made plus refined wheat, white bread, and so on.

Trans fats: Found in margarine and distinctive dealt with sustenance.

Oils that are refined: Canola oil, soybean oil, cottonseed oil, etc.

Taken care of meat: Processed sausages, wieners, etc.

Significantly took care of sustenance: Anything named "low-fat" or "diet" or which appears like it was made in a creation line.

You ought to scrutinize food checks mindfully if you have to avoid these unfortunate trimmings.

Nutrition to Eat

The eating routine examined by most examinations is high in strong plant sustenance and modestly low in animal food sources.

Regardless, eating fish and fish is recommended in any occasion multiple times each week.

The Mediterranean lifestyle similarly incorporates standard physical activity, offering suppers to other people and acknowledging life.

You should assemble your eating routine as for this strong, characteristic Mediterranean sustenance:

-Vegetables: Tomatoes, broccoli, kale, spinach, onions, cauliflower, carrots, Brussels fledglings, cucumbers, etc.

-Regular items: Apples, bananas, oranges, pears, strawberries, grapes, dates, figs, melons, peaches, etc.

-Nuts as well as seeds: Walnuts, almonds, macadamia nuts, cashews, and hazelnuts seeds, sunflower pumpkin seeds, and so on.

-Vegetables: Beans, peas, lentils, beats, peanuts, chickpeas, etc.

-Tubers: Potatoes, sweet potatoes, turnips, yams, etc.

-Whole grains: Whole oats, hearty hued rice, rye, grain, corn, buckwheat, whole wheat, whole grain bread and pasta.

-Fish and fish: Salmon, sardines, trout, fish, mackerel, shrimp, shellfish, mollusks, crab, mussels, etc.

-Poultry: Chicken, duck, turkey, etc.

-Eggs: Chicken, quail and duck eggs.

-Dairy: Cheese, yogurt, Greek yogurt, etc.

-Flavors and flavors: Garlic, basil, mint, rosemary, sage, nutmeg, cinnamon, pepper, etc.

-Sound Fats: Extra virgin olive oil, olives, avocados and avocado oil.

-Whole, single-fixing sustenance are the best approach to incredible prosperity.

What to Drink

Water should be your go-to reward on a Mediterranean eating schedule.

This eating routine furthermore joins moderate proportions of red wine — around 1 glass for stated timing.

Regardless, this is absolutely optional, and wine should be dodged by anyone with alcohol misuse or issues controlling their usage.

Coffee and tea are moreover absolutely commendable, yet you should avoid sugar-improved rewards and natural item squeezes, which are high in sugar.

CHAPTER THREE

MEDITERRANEAN MEAL PLAN FOR ONE WHOLE WEEK PLUS MUNCHIES FOR YOU

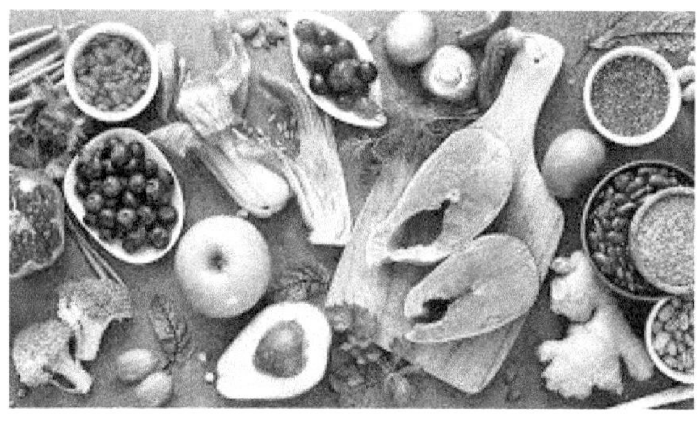

A Mediterranean Delicious Sample Menu for 1 whole Week

Coming up next is a model menu for multi week on the Mediterranean eating routine.

Try not to spare a moment to adjust the sections and food choices subject to your own needs and tendencies.

Monday

Breakfast: Greek yogurt plus strawberries as well as oats.

Lunch: Whole grain sandwich as well as vegetables.

Dinner: A fish bowl of combined greens, wearing olive oil. A touch of typical item for dessert.

Tuesday

Breakfast: Oatmeal with raisins.

Lunch: Leftover fish plate of blended greens from the earlier night.

Dinner: Salad with tomatoes, olives and feta cheddar.

Wednesday

Breakfast: Omelet with veggies, tomatoes plus onions. A touch of characteristic item.

Lunch: Whole grain sandwich plus cheddar as well as new vegetables.

Dinner: Mediterranean lasagne.

Thursday

Breakfast: Yogurt plus cut results of the dirt.

Lunch: Leftover lasagne from the earlier night.

Dinner: Broiled salmon, given gritty hued rice plus vegetables.

Friday

Breakfast: Eggs plus vegetables, burned in olive oil.

Lunch: Greek yogurt plus strawberries, oats as well as nuts.

Dinner: Grilled sheep, with plate of blended greens and warmed potato.

Saturday

Breakfast: Oatmeal plus raisins, nuts as well as an apple.

Lunch: Whole grain sandwich plus vegetables.

Dinner: Mediterranean pizza made with whole wheat, polished off with cheddar, vegetables plus olives.

Sunday

Breakfast: Omelet plus veggies as well as olives.

Lunch: Leftover pizza from the earlier night.

Dinner: Grilled chicken plus vegetables as well as a potato. Characteristic item for dessert.

There is typically no convincing motivation to check calories or track macronutrients (protein, fat and carbs) on the Mediterranean eating routine.

Strong Mediterranean munchies

You don't need to eat various dinners consistently.

However, in case you become hungry between dinners, there are a ton of strong snack decisions:

-An unassuming pack of nuts.

-A touch of natural item.

-Carrots or baby carrots.

-A couple of berries or grapes.

-Additional items from the earlier night.

-Greek yogurt.

-Apple cuts with almond margarine.

Bit by bit directions to follow the Diet at
Restaurants

It's anything but difficult to make most bistro
suppers proper for the Mediterranean eating
routine.

Pick fish or fish as your crucial dish.

Solicitation that they fry your food in extra virgin
olive oil.

Simply eat whole grain bread, with olive oil
instead of spread.

It is reliably a brilliant idea to shop at the outskirt of the store. That is normally where the whole sustenance is.

Consistently endeavor to pick the least-took care of decision. Characteristic is ideal, yet just if you can without a very remarkable stretch deal with its expense.

Vegetables: Carrots, onions, broccoli, spinach, kale, garlic, etc.

Natural items: Apples, bananas, oranges, grapes, etc.

Berries: Strawberries, blueberries, etc.

Hardened veggies: Choose mixes in with sound vegetables.

Grains: Whole-grain bread, whole grain pasta, etc.

Vegetables: Lentils, beats, beans, etc.

Nuts: Almonds, walnuts, cashews, etc.

Seeds: Sunflower seeds, pumpkin seeds, etc.

Trimmings: Sea salt, pepper, turmeric, cinnamon, etc.

Fish: Salmon, sardines, mackerel, trout.

-Shrimp and shellfish.

-Potatoes and sweet potatoes.

-Cheddar.

-Greek yogurt.

-Chicken.

-Taken care of or omega-3 improved eggs.

-Olives.

-Extra virgin olive oil.

It's ideal to clear all sad temptations from your home, including soda pops, solidified yogurt, candy, prepared products, white bread, and saltines should be dealt with sustenance.

If you simply have sound food in your home, guarantee you eat well.

CHAPTER FOUR

MOTIVATIONS TO HELP YOU FALL IN LOVEWITH THE MEDITERRANEAN DIET

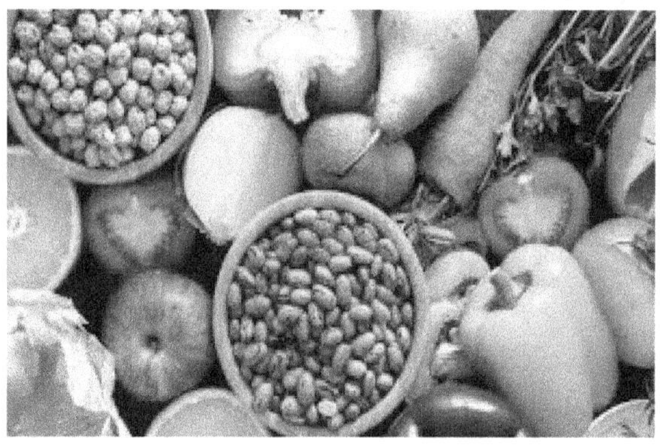

i. No Calorie Counting

Olive oil sprinkled over bread

You won't need a mini-computer for this supper plan. Rather than including numbers, you trade out terrible fats for heart-sound ones. Go for olive oil rather than spread. Make do with poultry or fishas a substitute for red meat. Appreciate new foods grown from the ground sweet, extravagant treats.

Eat your fill of tasty veggies and beans. Nuts are acceptable, yet adhere to a small bunch a day. You can have entire grain bread and wine, yet in moderate sums.

ii. The Food Is Really Fresh

Greek plate of mixed greens

You won't have to wander the solidified food passageway or hit an inexpensive food drive-through. The emphasis is on occasional food that is made in straightforward, mouth-watering ways. Manufacture a yummy plate of mixed greens from spinach, cucumbers, and tomatoes. Include exemplary Greek fixings like dark olives and feta cheddar with a Quick Light Greek Salad formula. You can likewise prepare a bright, veggie-filled clump of Grilled Tomato Gazpacho.

iii. You Can Have Bread

Grape and apple sandwich in wholegrain pita

Search for a portion made with entire grains. It has more protein and minerals and is commonly more advantageous than the white flour kind. Attempt entire grain pita bread plunged in olive oil, hummus, or tahini (a protein-rich glue produced using ground sesame seeds).

iv. Fat Isn't Forbidden

Pesto in bowl

You simply need to search for the great kind.
You'll see it in nuts, olives, and olive oil. These
fats (not the immersed and trans fat covered up
in prepared nourishments) include flavor and
help battle maladies from diabetes to
malignancy. Fundamental Basil Pesto is a
delectable method to get some into your eating
routine.

v. The Menu Is Huge

Moroccan tangines

It's something beyond Greek and Italian food.
You can perhaps look for plans from Turkey,
Morocco, Spain as well as different nations. Pick
nourishments that adhere to the essentials: light
on red meat and entire fat dairy, with bunches of
new foods grown from the ground, olive oil, and
entire grains. This Moroccan plan plus chickpeas,

flavors, okra and suits the solid Mediterranean profile.

vi. The Spices Are Delicious

Cod with rosemary

Straight leaves, cilantro, coriander, rosemary, garlic, pepper, and cinnamon include so many flavors you won't have to go after the salt shaker. Some have medical advantages, as well. Coriander and rosemary, for instance, have ailment battling cancer prevention agents and supplements. This formula for Greek-Style Mushrooms utilizes cilantro and coriander and has a lemony kick.

vii. It's Easy to Make

Little plates of olives and cheddar

Greek suppers are frequently little, simple to gather plates called mezzes. For your own serve-it-cold easygoing supper, you could put out plates of cheddar, olives, and nuts. Additionally look at these plans for Basil Quinoa With Red Bell Pepper and Eight Layered Greek Dip. Both have heart-accommodating fixings including olive oil, beans, entire grains, and flavors.

viii. You Can Have Wine

Companions appreciating wine (red) with supper.

A glass with suppers is regular in numerous Mediterranean nations, where feasting is frequently comfortable and social. A few examinations recommend that for certain individuals, up to one glass a day for ladies and two for men might be useful for your heart.

ix. You Won't Be Hungry

Bowls of hummus and bean plunges

You'll get an opportunity to eat rich-tasting nourishments like cooked yams, hummus, and even this Lima Bean Spread. You digest them gradually with the goal that you feel full more. Yearning's not an issue when you can chomp on nuts, olives, or nibbles of low-fat cheddar when a hankering strikes. Feta and halloumi are lower in fat than cheddar yet rich and delicious.

x. You Can Lose Weight

Man remaining on scale

You'd figure it would take a wonder to drop a few pounds in the event that you eat nuts, cheddar, and oils. Yet, those Mediterranean fundamentals (and the more slow eating style) let you feel full and fulfilled. Also, that causes you adhere to an eating routine. Normal exercise is additionally a significant aspect of the way of life.

xi. Your Heart Will Thank You

Avocados loaded down with fish and vegetables.

Nearly everything in this eating regimen is useful for your heart. Olive oil and nuts assistance lower "terrible" cholesterol. Organic products, veggies, and beans help keep veins clear. Fish helps lower fatty substances and circulatory strain. In the event that you've never gone gaga for fish, attempt this Mediterranean-enlivened formula for Grilled Whole Trout With Lemon-Tarragon Bean Salad.

xii. You'll Stay Sharper and Longer

Brilliant slashed chime peppers.

A similar goodness that ensures your heart is likewise useful for your mind. You're not eating terrible fats and handled nourishments, which can cause aggravation. Rather, cancer prevention agent rich nourishments make this eating style a mind benevolent decision.

CHAPTER FIVE

MEDITERRANEAN DIET VERSUS DIFFERENT DIETS: WHICH IS PERFECT?

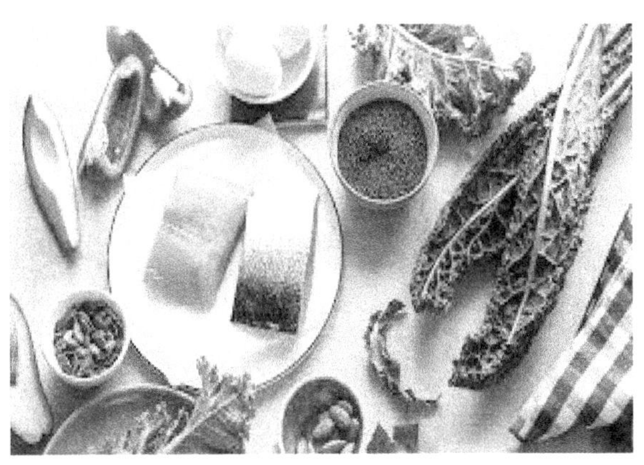

In case you're as of now investigating diets to attempt, you presumably unearthed a huge amount of alternatives.

Remember there's nobody diet that works for everybody. While looking for the correct eating routine, it's imperative to pick something that works for your way of life, that advances great wellbeing, and that is practical to adhere to long haul.

The Mediterranean eating regimen is a very much explored eating plan that may mark off these measures for some individuals. This eating regimen unmistakably covers with most USDA Dietary Guidelines, maybe with a couple of extra details, and offers a few focal points contrasted with other well-known diets.

The 2019 U.S. News and World Report Best Diets position the Mediterranean Diet number 1 in Best Diets Overall and gives it a general score of 4.2/5.

USDA Recommendations For You

The Mediterranean eating routine is very like the USDA Dietary Guidelines, except for a couple of somewhat stricter rules.

Nutrition classes

The Mediterranean eating regimen incorporates each of the five nutritional categories that are available in the USDA Guidelines. These incorporate natural products, vegetables, protein, dairy, and grains.

The Mediterranean eating regimen offers extra rules inside a portion of these gatherings, however. For instance, while the USDA suggests in any event a large portion of your grains originate from entire grains; the Mediterranean eating routine suggests that all grains are entire grains (except for infrequent suppers).

Also, while the USDA treats a wide range of protein similarly, the Mediterranean eating regimen indicates that specific proteins, similar to red meat, should just be expended every so often. Other creature proteins ought to be utilized in littler parts too.

These distinctions are not excessively prohibitive, however may demonstrate troublesome if your present eating routine is a long way from meeting the rules.

Calories

There is no particular number of calories suggested on the Mediterranean eating regimen. Since it's an eating design instead of an organized eating routine, the attention is on great, supplement thick nourishments, as opposed to tallying calories.

All things considered, calorie balance is as yet a key factor in weight the board. You can discover USDA Guidelines for calories dependent on age, tallness, sexual orientation, and action level. You can likewise take a stab at utilizing our calorie objective mini-computer to get a gauge. These calorie levels can undoubtedly be applied inside the structure of a Mediterranean style diet.

In case you're following the Mediterranean eating routine yet end up putting on weight, take a stab at following your calorie consumption for a couple of days to check whether it's similar to these suggestions. Make little changes to alter as fundamental.

Assortment

An accentuation on assortment! Both supper arranging approaches urge you to incorporate an assortment of produce and stir up your decisions normally.

For instance, do you generally stay with an icy mass lettuce side serving of mixed greens? Take a stab at switching things up with romaine, spinach, arugula, or another verdant green.

Is your go-to side at supper a pack of solidified broccoli? Take a stab at snatching an alternate solidified veggie at the store, or consider better approaches to get ready broccoli-like broiling it or making a soup.

Not exclusively will this guarantee you're meeting your dietary needs, yet it will likewise grow your sense of taste and make supper time more fun.

Comparable Diets

The Mediterranean eating routine offers comparable highlights to other mainstream eats less carbs however offers more adaptability than most. It's likewise incredibly all around investigated, which is extraordinary for some, famous eating routine plans. Here's a speedy breakdown of how it looks at.

Mediterranean Diet

General nourishment: This eating regimen is wealthy in plant-based segments like organic products, vegetables, entire grains, and olive oil. It incorporates all nourishments; however it determines that red meat and included sugar should just be utilized not very often. When followed, it ought to be anything but difficult to meet your supplement needs.

Medical advantages: Perhaps the most investigated of any eating routine; it is related with a lower danger of coronary illness, malignant growth, and other constant diseases.

Weight reduction: The Mediterranean eating regimen has been found to help with weight reduction and weight the board—despite the fact that it is high in calorie-thick nourishments like olive oil and nuts.

Maintainability: This eating regimen is solid and possible to follow forever. In case you're a substantial red meat eater you may battle, however even an adjusted variant with higher measures of red meat has been appeared to improve wellbeing markers.

Flexitarian Diet

General sustenance: The Flexitarian diet
(otherwise called an adaptable veggie lover)
incorporates all nutritional categories however
suggests restricting creature proteins. It is
fundamentally the same as the Mediterranean
eating routine, accentuating heaps of produce,
entire grains, and sound oils.

Medical advantages: Studies have connected a
Flexitarian diet to bring down danger of diabetes,
and the reasonable idea of the eating routine
probably has other ceaseless illness counteraction
benefits.

Weight reduction: Several examinations have
demonstrated that semi-veggie lover eats less,
similar to the flexitarian diet, are related with
lower body weight or BMI.

Maintainability: Just like the Mediterranean eating routine, the vast majority ought to have the option to tail it long haul. In the event that you appreciate high measures of creature items you may battle, yet the arrangement is very adaptable to take into consideration tailing it such that works for you.

Keto Diet

General nourishment: While many think about the Mediterranean eating routine similar to a higher fat eating regimen (around 35-40 percent, because of high olive oil and nut utilization), the keto diet contains undeniably more fat (roughly 75 percent). The keto diet additionally seriously restricts sugars, which means nourishments like entire grains, vegetables, and most organic products are beyond reach. These serious limitations can make it hard to address dietary issues.

Medical advantages: The keto diet's viability is settled for epilepsy.6 However, for other ailments, the advantages stay questionable. For individuals with certain ailments, similar to pregnancy or type 1 diabetes, it can really be hazardous to begin a keto diet.

Weight reduction: Several investigations have demonstrated that a ketogenic diet assists patients with getting thinner. One efficient audit found that at one year, those on a keto style diet shed around 4 pounds more than those on a low-fat diet. However, there is minimal long haul research on these results.

Supportability: You may discover it very testing to stay with the keto diet long haul, as it's unquestionably more prohibitive than something like the Mediterranean eating regimen.

DASH/Run Diet

General sustenance: The DASH diet, all the more
officially known as Dietary Approaches to Stop
Hypertension, depends on eating principally
natural products, vegetables, low-fat dairy, entire
grains, and bit controlled lean protein. A portion
of these proposals are like the Mediterranean
eating regimen (i.e bunches of produce), however
DASH places more prominent accentuation on
low-fat dairy and protein. There is additionally a
sodium limit.

Medical advantages: Research has indicated the
DASH diet brings down circulatory strain and
improves cholesterol.

Weight reduction: A 2016 survey carried out
about DASH diet, revealed that this diet
advanced weight reduction and improved BMI.
Calorie-controlled DASH eats less carbs
prompted considerably more noteworthy results.

Maintainability: The DASH diet is another eating regimen, similar to the Mediterranean eating routine that can be plausible to follow forever. Be that as it may, it requires all the more wanting to meet explicit nutrition type servings and sodium limitations, which may demonstrate trying for the individuals who aren't exceptionally energetic.

CHAPTER SIX

THE HEALTH GAINS OF MEDITERRANEAN DIET; FOR WEIGHT LOSS PLUS THE REASON FOR BEING A PERFECT DIET AND OTHER FACTS

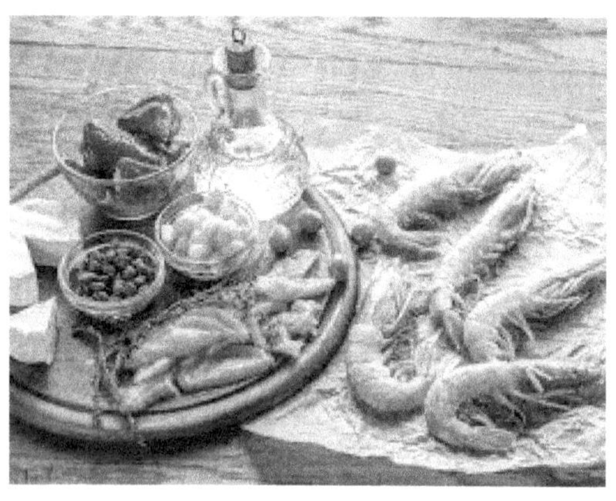

Each culture has its own interpretation of what makes a sound eating regimen. Frequently the varieties between cooking styles of various areas depends on what's locally accessible. For instance, the corn that America is so notable for isn't developed in all sides of the world, while the chickpeas and olives that give Middle Eastern dishes their unmistakable pizazz might be less generally accessible in different pieces of the world.

Two territorially motivated ways to deal with good dieting have taken the jump toward formal, conspicuous weight control plans. The Mediterranean eating routine, which approximates the dietary propensities for individuals living close to the Mediterranean Sea, and the Nordic eating regimen, which imitates wellbeing cognizant, current Scandinavian way to deal with food and way of life, are presently viewed as great choices for individuals all over the place.

Mediterranean Diet Overview

The Mediterranean eating regimen has been a most loved of dietitians the world over for a long time. Created during the 1960s as methods for lessening the frequency of coronary illness, the Mediterranean eating routine obtains numerous chiefs of eating from a few southern European nations.

The Mediterranean eating regimen supports utilization of entire grains as well as vegetables, which are significant wellsprings of fiber in our eating routine.

It additionally incorporates loads of heart-solid olive oil. Cheeses, especially those produced using sheep's or goat's milk –, for example, feta, chevre and pecorino – are utilized in numerous Mediterranean dishes. Yogurt, explicitly thick, velvety Greek yogurt, is additionally important for the eating routine.

The Mediterranean eating routine is about balance and is an example of eating, instead of a prohibitive eating regimen. Thusly, no food is untouchable, yet dairy, red meat, desserts and handled nourishments are devoured in littler amounts, the study reveals.

Nordic Diet Overview

Like the Mediterranean eating regimen, the Nordic eating routine acquires eating standards from individuals living in one area, explicitly the Nordic nations of Denmark, Finland, Iceland, Norway and Sweden.

The Nordic eating regimen favors a plant-first methodology that likewise incorporates moderate measures of fish and eggs and some dairy items. Since the accentuation is on utilizing privately sourced and reasonably gathered produce, the fish highlighted in the Nordic eating routine will in general be the greasy, cold-water fish indigenous to the district – herring, mackerel, salmon and sardines. These fish are high in heart-sound omega-3 unsaturated fats.

You may likewise observe a sprinkling of matured and salted nourishments on the Nordic eating routine, for example, yogurt and kefir, cured herring and cured vegetables. Aged nourishments help uphold a sound stomach related framework.

Since it stresses neighborhood, in-season produce, the Nordic eating regimen may likewise be preferred for the earth over the standard American eating routine, which will in general support handled nourishments and all year accessibility of most products of the soil. **Development of red meat has additionally been connected to natural concerns, so counts calories that incorporate less of these nourishments might be better for the planet.**

The standard American eating regimen is additionally ordinarily substantial in salt and handled nourishments. A plant-based methodology can take out a portion of those issues.

The greatest contrast between the Mediterranean and Nordic weight control plans comes in the kind of oil utilized. While the Mediterranean eating regimen favors locally-accessible and ample olive oil, olives aren't in wealth in Nordic nations. Consequently, rapeseed oil, otherwise called canola oil, is the essential fat source. Canola oil offers comparative medical advantages to olive oil, and it's been related with improved cardiovascular wellbeing.

Medical advantages

Mediterranean eating routine. Various investigations and audits have been distributed indicating benefits for diabetes; cardiovascular wellbeing including stroke counteraction, as well as restricted information connecting the Mediterranean eating routine to the anticipation of Alzheimer's and misery says modern research. Diminished danger and better administration of Type 2 diabetes has additionally been related with the Mediterranean eating regimen. Since it's high in fiber and lessens admission of handled and red meats, the Mediterranean eating regimen is likewise connected with a decreased danger of colon disease.

Nordic eating routine. The new Nordic eating regimen is a fresher methodology, with the standards being built up in 2004 by a gathering of nourishing researchers situated in Copenhagen, Denmark. Yet, it has its foundations in conventional Scandinavian dietary propensities. Since the eating routine is generally new, it hasn't been concentrated as widely as more seasoned conventions like the Mediterranean eating regimen, however it follows comparable standards, and the medical advantages are believed to be comparative.

Reasonably developed, privately sourced products of the soil structure the foundation of the eating regimen. These nourishments give heaps of fiber, nutrients and supplements that are essential to acceptable wellbeing. The consideration of sound fats and greasy fish, for example, herring and salmon, that are rich wellsprings of omega-3 unsaturated fats can likewise improve in general wellbeing, decrease frequency of Type 2 diabetes and lessen danger of particular kinds of malignancy and other constant infections. Search for more exploration soon as studies into the eating regimen's medical advantages increment.

Since both the Mediterranean and Nordic eating regimens stress plant-based wellsprings of sustenance, they can be an incredible option in contrast to different methods of eating.

Natural products, vegetables, entire grains, vegetables, nuts and seeds, you are successfully lessening calorie utilization, which can help with weight reduction as well as sound weight support. That, thusly, can decrease heftiness, a contributing variable to numerous interminable sicknesses.

Furthermore, plant-based nourishments are supplement thick, which means they have a larger number of supplements for their weight than the proportional load of prepared or quick nourishments. Expanding plant-based nourishments additionally builds nutrients and minerals, just as cancer prevention agents, which are valuable for wellbeing and shirking of ceaseless illness the study reveals.

Wellbeing Risks

Mediterranean eating routine; no particular wellbeing chances are known to be connected to the Mediterranean eating routine the study reveals. Yet, it takes note of that in certain translations, moderate measures of red wine might be incorporated, as well as liquor utilization isn't proper for everybody

Nordic eating routine; scarcely any particular wellbeing hazards have been related with the Nordic eating regimen. All things considered, changing how you eat can adjust your admission of specific supplements, so it's ideal to look for the exhortation of an enlisted dietitian or other wholesome master before you drastically change what you're eating.

In spite of the fact that an expanded admission of specific kinds of fish can build levels of mercury that could have wellbeing impacts, the littler the fish, ordinarily the less mercury it has in its body. Since a significant part of the fish on the Nordic eating routine are littler in size and in this way lower on the natural pecking order, they tend not to have as much mercury pollution as bigger fish, for example, fish or swordfish. Sardines, anchovies, herring and salmon are completely viewed as better fish alternatives. What's more, since fish isn't eaten each day on the Nordic eating routine, mercury harming is definitely not a significant concern.

Expenses

The study says the Mediterranean eating regimen can be followed on a tight spending plan, and that working with an enrolled dietitian can assist you with discovering more prudent approaches to staying with the arrangement. Beans, lentils and mass entire grains are the absolute most affordable things in the supermarket, so consumes fewer calories that depend on these might be helpful.

Since the Nordic eating routine courtesies natural produce, it could be somewhat pricier than some different alternatives out there. In any case, in the event that you decide on customarily developed produce instead of just purchasing natural foods grown from the ground that could chop down your staple bill.

Weight reduction

The two eating regimens can be acceptable decisions in case you're attempting to get more fit. Be that as it may, you have to hold parcels under tight restraints. It's completely conceivable to put on weight on either diet in case you're eating an excess of food.

The Mediterranean eating regimen tied for seventeenth spot on U.S. News' Best Weight-Loss Diets in 2019. A recent report in the diary Nutrition and Diabetes found that the Mediterranean eating routine was related with lower levels of weight gain and a lower increment in midriff periphery over the 12-year range of the investigation.

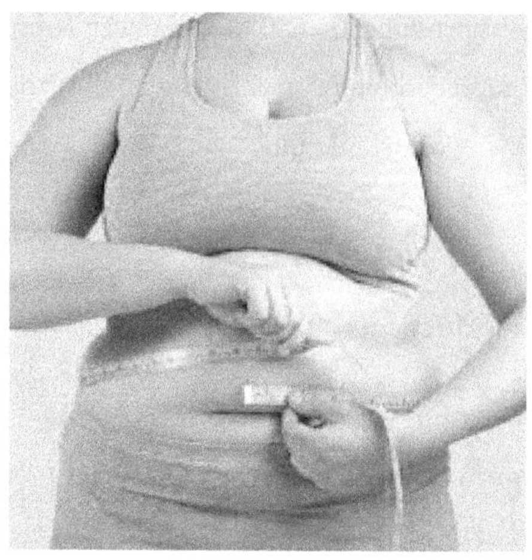

The Nordic eating routine tied for 26th spot in the 2019 best weight reduction positioning. As per a recent studies that contrasted the new Nordic eating routine with a normal Danish eating regimen (which like the standard American eating routine is higher in fat, sugar, meat and prepared nourishments), members on

the Nordic eating regimen were bound to shed
pounds. Studies are continuous, yet once more,
balance and segment control are the way to
getting in shape with most or any eating routine
– the Nordic eating regimen included.

Why it is a Perfect Diet?

The Mediterranean eating regimen has reliably
positioned No. 1 generally speaking in U.S. News'
Best Diets rankings. In 2019, the Nordic eating
routine tied for ninth in general.

These two eating regimens are fundamentally the
same as far as medical advantages, dangers,
expenses and weight reduction, so the assurance
of which is better generally comes down to taste.
Do you lean toward the olive-based kinds of
southern Europe? Or on the other hand do you
like a more Scandinavian energy to your dishes?

The choice is yours; since your very choice is
centered on your preference for a particular diet.

CHAPTER SEVEN

CONCLUSION

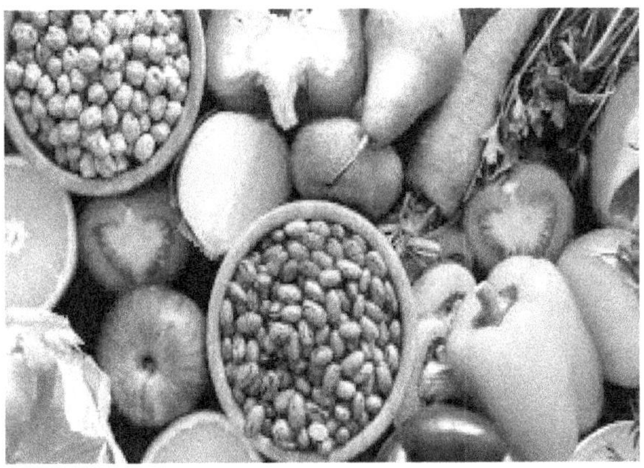

In spite of the fact that there isn't one characterized Mediterranean eating regimen, this method of eating is commonly wealthy in sound plant nourishments and generally lower in creature food sources, with an attention on fish.

Toward the day's end, the Mediterranean eating routine is inconceivably sound and fulfilling. You won't be frustrated. I tell you!

Lastly, you are sure to get the expected results when the guidelines as well as the secrets in this guide are strictly followed. Best of luck to you as you begin your **Mediterranean** diets preparation!

THE END

www.ingramcontent.com/pod-product-compliance
Lightning Source LLC
Chambersburg PA
CBHW071447150726
48000CB00006B/2469